COMPLETE GUIDE TO UNDERSTANDING HIP REPLACEMENT SURGERY

Expert Insights To Procedures, Recovery, Rehabilitation, Surgical Techniques, Postoperative Care, And More

KLEIN HOYLE

© [KLEIN HOYLE] [2024]

All rights reserved.

No part of this book may be reproduced, distributed, or transmitted in any form or by any means, including photocopying, recording, or other electronic or mechanical methods, without the publisher's prior written permission, with the exception of brief quotations in critical reviews and certain other noncommercial uses permitted by copyright law.

Disclaimer

The content in this book is based on the author's expertise and comprehension of the topic. The author has no affiliation or link with any corporation, business, or person. This book is meant to give general information and educational material only, and it should not be interpreted as professional medical advice. Always seek the advice of a skilled healthcare expert if you have any queries about medical issues or treatments. The author and publisher expressly disclaim any responsibility resulting directly or indirectly from the use or use of the information included in this book.

Table of Contents

CHAPTER 1 15
- Introduction To Hip Replacement Surgery 15
- What Is Hip Replacement Surgery? 15
- When Is Hip Replacement Surgery Necessary? ... 16
  - 2. Loss of Mobility: 16
  - 3. Joint Damage: 16
  - 4. Conservative Treatment Failure: 17
- Types Of Hip Replacement Surgery 17
  - 2. Partial Hip Replacement (Hemiarthroplasty): 17
  - 3. Minimally Invasive Hip Replacement: 18
  - 4. Revision Hip Replacement: 18
- Overview Of The Procedure 18

CHAPTER 2 21
- Understanding Hip Anatomy 21
- Basics Of Hip Anatomy 21
- Common Hip Problems And Conditions 22
- How Does Hip Replacement Surgery Address These Issues? 23
- Preparing For Surgery: Knowing Your Hip Condition 24

CHAPTER 3 27
  Preparing For Surgery 27
  Pre-Operative Assessment And Testing 27
  Meet With Your Surgeon And Medical Team....28
  Preparing Your Home For Post-Surgical Recovery
 29
  Pre-Operative Workouts And Physical Therapy.30
CHAPTER 4 33
  The Surgical Process 33
  Anesthesia Options For Hip Replacement Surgery
 33
    2. Regional Anesthesia:................................34
    3. Combination anesthetic: 34
  A Step-By-Step Overview Of The Surgical
  Procedure...35
    1. Preparation:...35
    3. Damaged Tissue Removal:......................36
    4. Implant placement: 36
    5. Closure: 36
  Potential Risks And Complications 37
    1. Infection: 37

    2. Blood Clots: 37

    3. Dislocation: 38

    4. Implant Wear and Loosening: 38

Post-Surgical Recovery In The Hospital 38

    1. Pain Management: 39

    2. Physical Therapy: 39

    3. Monitoring: 39

    4. Diet and Hydration: 39

    5. Discharge Planning: 40

CHAPTER 5 41

Post-Surgical Recovery 41

Pain Management Techniques 41

Physical Therapy Exercises For Recovery 42

Managing Daily Activities Throughout Recovery 44

Potential Complications And How To Manage Them 46

CHAPTER 6 49

Rehabilitation And Physical Therapy 49

Importance Of Rehabilitation Following Hip Replacement Surgery 49

Schedule For Rehabilitation Exercises 50
Exercises To Increase Strength And Mobility 52
   1. Hip Flexion: 53
   2. Hip Extension: 53
   3. Hip abduction: 53
   4. Hip Adduction: 54
   5. Quadriceps Strengthening: 54
   6. Core Strengthening: 54
Tips For A Successful Rehabilitation Process 55
   1. Follow the Rehabilitation Program: 55
   2. Take it Slow: 55
   3. Stay Active: 55
   4. Use Assistive Devices as Needed: 55
   5. Practice Good Posture and Body Mechanics: 56
   6. Maintain a positive attitude: 56
CHAPTER 7 57
  Returning To Daily Activities 57
  Gradual Resumption Of Daily Activity 57
  Modifications For Activities Such As Driving And 58

    Guidelines For Physical Activity And Exercise ..59

    Long-Term Expectations For Hip Function.......60

CHAPTER 8 61

    Complications And Risks...............................61

    Common Complications Following Hip Replacement Surgery 61

    Symptoms Of An Infection Or Other Complications..64

    Steps To Take If Complications Arise 66

    Strategies To Prevent Complications...............68

CHAPTER 9 71

    Lifestyle Modifications.................................71

    Recommendations To Maintain Hip Health 71

    Dietary Considerations For Bone Health..........73

    Exercise And Activity Guidelines For Long-Term Hip Health 74

    Tips To Prevent Future Hip Problems 76

CHAPTER 10 79

    Moving Forward..79

    Recap Of Key Points On Hip Replacement Surgery 79

        Understanding the Surgery: 79

    Preoperative Preparations: 80

    Surgical Procedure: 80

    Postoperative Care: 80

Encouragement To Continue Recovery And Rehabilitation 81

    Stay Active: 81

    Follow Medical Advice: 82

    Manage Expectations: 82

    Seek help: 82

Looking Ahead: Life Following Hip Replacement Surgery 83

    Regaining Independence: 83

    Returning to Activities: 83

    Embracing a Healthy Lifestyle: 84

    Staying Informed: 84

    Enjoying Life: 84

Conclusion 85

THE END 89

ABOUT THIS BOOK

The "Complete Guide to Understanding Hip Replacement Surgery" is a great resource for anyone dealing with the intricacies of hip replacement surgery. This book, with its full treatment of the surgical technique and intelligent talks on pre and post-surgery care, is a beacon of information and support for patients and their caregivers.

Chapter 1 introduces readers to the principles of hip replacement surgery, including indications, types, and an overview of the operation. This fundamental information builds the foundations for comprehending the future chapters, offering clarity and perspective for the trip ahead.

Chapter 2 goes into the complexities of hip anatomy, describing prevalent hip disorders and how hip replacement surgery solves them. Understanding one's hip condition is critical for making educated decisions and achieving the best results, therefore this chapter serves as an excellent beginning point for readers.

Preparation is essential, and Chapter 3 walks readers through the pre-surgery procedure, from examinations and testing to preparing their house for recuperation. Patients who are well-prepared for surgery may approach their procedure with confidence and peace of mind.

The surgical method is fully examined in Chapter 4, which includes anesthetic alternatives, step-by-step procedural information, and possible risks and consequences. This thorough awareness enables individuals to actively participate in their treatment and work successfully with their medical team.

Post-surgery recovery, as described in Chapter 5, is a key period that requires careful pain management, attention to physical therapy exercises, and watching for complications.

This chapter makes the transition from surgery to therapy more manageable by giving practical solutions and insights.

Chapter 6 stresses the significance of rehabilitation and physical therapy in regaining hip function and mobility. Patients may confidently and resolutely pursue their rehabilitation path with a defined timeframe and workout instructions.

Returning to everyday activities, as outlined in Chapter 7, is an important milestone in the rehabilitation process. Readers are given suggestions for gradually resuming activities, making required changes, and ensuring long-term hip health.

Chapters 8 and 9 discuss probable problems and lifestyle changes, allowing readers to reduce risks and improve general well-being after surgery. Patients who adopt preventative measures and healthy practices may improve their results and quality of life.

Chapter 10 encourages readers to reflect on their experiences, celebrate milestones, and approach life following hip replacement surgery with hope and perseverance. This last chapter acts as a light of hope, encouraging readers to continue their road to recovery and well-being.

CHAPTER 1

Introduction To Hip Replacement Surgery

What Is Hip Replacement Surgery?

Hip replacement surgery, also known as hip arthroplasty, is a surgical operation used to replace a broken or diseased hip joint with an artificial implant. This technique is often used when other therapies, such as drugs, physical therapy, or lifestyle changes, have failed to alleviate hip discomfort and mobility difficulties.

The hip joint is a ball-and-socket joint, with the ball-shaped head of the femur (thigh bone) fitting into the socket-shaped acetabulum of the pelvis. Over time, the cartilage that lines the surfaces of these bones may degrade owing to illnesses such as osteoarthritis, rheumatoid arthritis, avascular necrosis, or injury, resulting in discomfort, stiffness, and limited mobility.

Hip replacement surgery tries to address these symptoms by replacing the damaged joint surfaces with prosthetic devices.

When Is Hip Replacement Surgery Necessary?

When conservative therapy fails to alleviate hip pain and impairment, a healthcare provider may prescribe hip replacement surgery. Common indications for hip replacement surgery are:

1. Severe hip pain is chronic and debilitating, limiting everyday activities and lowering quality of life.

2. **Loss of Mobility:** Difficulties walking, climbing stairs, or doing normal duties owing to hip stiffness and limited range of motion.

3. **Joint Damage:** Significant degradation of the hip joint caused by arthritis, injury, or other degenerative disorders, as detected by imaging examinations such as X-rays or MRIs.

4. Conservative Treatment Failure: Inadequate pain and symptom alleviation despite the use of drugs, physical therapy, corticosteroid injections, or assistive aids such as canes or walkers.

Types Of Hip Replacement Surgery

Hip replacement procedures are classified into numerous categories, each of which is intended to meet distinct patient demands and conditions:

1. The most frequent kind of hip replacement surgery is total hip replacement (THR), which involves replacing both the ball and socket of the hip joint with prosthetic components composed of metal, plastic, or ceramic materials.

2. Partial Hip Replacement (Hemiarthroplasty): During this treatment, just the ball of the hip joint is replaced with a prosthetic component, leaving the socket intact. This method is often utilized for individuals with certain kinds of hip fractures.

3. Minimally Invasive Hip Replacement: This approach uses fewer incisions and specialized devices, perhaps resulting in shorter recovery periods and less postoperative discomfort than typical hip replacement surgery.

4. Revision Hip Replacement: If a prior hip replacement fails due to infection, loosening, or wear and tear on the prosthetic components, a revision operation may be required to replace or repair the existing implants.

Overview Of The Procedure

Hip replacement surgery is often conducted using general anesthesia or regional anesthesia, in which just the lower half of the body is numbed. The surgical team will create an incision across the hip joint to expose the injured surfaces. The arthritic or diseased bone and cartilage are subsequently removed, and the prosthetic components are fixed in place using specialist bone cement or press-fit methods.

The innovative artificial joint is meant to mirror the hip's natural movement and function, resulting in smoother mobility and less discomfort. After the implants are installed, the incision is closed with sutures or staples, and a sterile dressing is given to the wound.

Pain management, physical therapy, and rehabilitation exercises are common postoperative treatments to help recover hip joint strength, flexibility, and mobility. Most patients should anticipate seeing a progressive improvement in their symptoms over many weeks to months after surgery, with complete recovery often occurring between 3 to 6 months.

Overall, hip replacement surgery may significantly relieve hip discomfort and restore mobility, enabling patients to resume regular daily activities and have a higher quality of life.

CHAPTER 2

Understanding Hip Anatomy

Basics Of Hip Anatomy

The hip is a wonder of engineering, with a ball-and-socket joint that provides both stability and movement. Imagine a golf ball lying on a tee: the ball represents the rounded head of the femur (thigh bone), and the tee represents the acetabulum, a cup-shaped socket in the pelvis. This configuration provides for a broad range of motion, which is essential for activities like walking, running, and even sitting.

Ligaments and muscles surround the hip joint, giving support and allowing for movement in several directions. The cartilage that covers the surfaces of the ball and socket lowers friction, resulting in smooth movement. A layer of synovial fluid inside the joint also lubricates and nourishes the cartilage, allowing for smooth mobility.

Common Hip Problems And Conditions

Despite its sturdy construction, the hip is prone to wear and strain, injury, and illness. Osteoarthritis, rheumatoid arthritis, avascular necrosis (loss of blood flow to the bone), hip fractures, and developmental dysplasia are some of the most common hip disorders.

Osteoarthritis, the most common hip condition, arises when the cartilage that cushions the joint breaks down over time, causing pain, stiffness, and limited mobility. Rheumatoid arthritis, an inflammatory illness, generates inflammation in the joint lining, which leads to pain, swelling, and, ultimately, joint deformity.

Hip fractures are common in elderly persons with weaker bones and may occur as a result of falls or accidents. Trauma or long-term steroid usage may cause avascular necrosis, which results in bone tissue death in the hip joint.

Developmental dysplasia typically affects babies, causing improper hip joint development and instability.

How Does Hip Replacement Surgery Address These Issues?

Hip replacement surgery, also known as total hip arthroplasty, is a life-changing technique that relieves pain and restores function in those who have significant hip issues. During surgery, the injured hip joint elements are replaced with prosthetic components composed of metal, plastic, or ceramic.

Hip replacement surgery for osteoarthritis and rheumatoid arthritis involves replacing worn-out cartilage and damaged bone with prosthetic components, therefore decreasing pain and enhancing mobility. Similarly, avascular necrosis and hip fractures are treated with surgery to replace the injured bone and restore joint stability.

By providing a smooth, lasting surface for the hip joint, the prosthetic components imitate the function of a healthy hip, enabling patients to reclaim their quality of life and participate in activities they like. Furthermore, advances in surgical methods and implant materials have considerably increased the lifetime and success rate of hip replacement surgeries.

Preparing For Surgery: Knowing Your Hip Condition

Preparing for hip replacement surgery entails a thorough examination of your hip condition and general health. Your orthopedic surgeon will do a comprehensive physical examination, examine your medical history, and may request imaging tests like X-rays or MRI scans to determine the amount of hip injury.

Understanding your hip health is critical for making educated treatment choices and establishing reasonable expectations for surgery.

Your surgeon will go over the risks and advantages of hip replacement, as well as other therapies including medication, physical therapy, and less invasive surgical procedures.

In addition to medical preparation, you may need to undertake lifestyle changes to improve your recovery and post-operative results. This might include maintaining a healthy weight, stopping smoking, and doing pre-operative exercises to strengthen the muscles around the hip joint.

By actively engaging in the preparation process and requesting advice from your healthcare team, you may guarantee a speedier recovery and the best potential outcomes following hip replacement surgery.

CHAPTER 3

Preparing For Surgery

Pre-Operative Assessment And Testing

Before hip replacement surgery, your medical team will undertake a comprehensive examination to verify you are physically fit for the operation. This examination consists of a battery of tests to check your general health, including blood tests, imaging scans, and perhaps an electrocardiogram (ECG) to measure heart function.

Blood tests are performed to rule out any underlying medical issues, such as infections or irregular blood clotting, that might jeopardize the operation or your recovery. Imaging studies, such as X-rays or MRIs, are used to determine the degree of damage to your hip joint and assist your surgeon in planning the operation.

An ECG may be conducted to assess your heart's electrical activity and guarantee that you may safely endure anesthesia and surgery. If any anomalies are found, more cardiac testing may be required before continuing with the hip replacement.

Meet With Your Surgeon And Medical Team

Once the pre-surgery examination is complete, you'll meet with your surgeon and medical team to go over the operation specifics and answer any concerns you may have. This is a crucial time to ask questions and make sure you understand what to anticipate before, during, and after surgery.

During this appointment, your surgeon will describe the surgical approach they want to utilize, the kind of implant to be used, and the possible risks and advantages of the surgery. They will also talk about any pre-existing medical issues you have and how they may affect the operation and recovery.

Your medical team will give you advice on how to prepare for the operation, including any medicines you must stop taking prior and any specific dietary requirements. They will also go over the various anesthetic alternatives and assist you in determining which one is appropriate for you based on your medical history and personal preferences.

Preparing Your Home For Post-Surgical Recovery

Preparing your house for post-surgical rehabilitation is critical to ensuring a smooth and pleasant recovery. Your medical staff will advise you on how to make your house safe and accessible for your reduced movement after surgery.

This might include rearranging furniture to provide clear routes for walking with crutches or a walker, putting handrails in restrooms and along stairs, and eliminating any tripping hazards like loose carpets or electrical cables.

If you usually sleep upstairs, you may want to set up a recuperation room on the first level of your house.

To handle pain and inflammation, you'll also need to stock up on vital goods like comfortable clothes, hygiene, and medicine. To ensure you have healthy food accessible throughout your recuperation period, plan ahead of time or arrange for meal delivery services.

Pre-Operative Workouts And Physical Therapy

In the weeks leading up to your hip replacement surgery, your doctor may advise you to do pre-operative exercises and physical therapy to strengthen the muscles around your hip joint and improve your general physical condition.

These exercises usually aim to improve flexibility, range of motion, and muscular strength in the hips, thighs, and core.

They might include mild stretches, low-impact aerobic activities like walking or swimming, and focused strength training exercises using resistance bands or small weights.

Physical therapy sessions may also be advised to teach you effective skills for utilizing assistive equipment like crutches or a walker, as well as pain and swelling management tactics after surgery. Participating in pre-operative exercises and physical therapy will help you enhance your physical condition and the result of hip replacement surgery.

CHAPTER 4

The Surgical Process

Anesthesia Options For Hip Replacement Surgery

When preparing for hip replacement surgery, one of the most important choices you and your medical team will make is the kind of anesthetic. There are various choices to examine, each with its own set of advantages and disadvantages.

1. General anesthesia is the most frequent kind of anesthetic used during hip replacement surgery. With general anesthesia, you will be fully asleep and ignorant of the surgery. It is delivered via an IV line or by breathing fumes via a mask. An anesthesiologist will continuously monitor your vital signs while you are under general anesthesia to guarantee your safety throughout the procedure.

2. Regional Anesthesia: Another alternative is regional anesthesia, which numbs a particular area of your body, in this instance, the lower half where the operation would be performed. There are two primary forms of regional anesthetic used during hip replacement surgery:

Spinal anesthesia involves injecting medicine into the spinal canal to numb the lower body from the waist down. This permits you to stay awake throughout the operation while experiencing no discomfort.

Epidural anesthesia, like spinal anesthesia, is administered by injecting medicine into the area around the spinal cord. It gives pain relief and muscular relaxation in the lower body, but it may also be utilized for long-term pain management after surgery.

3. Combination anesthetic: In certain situations, a combination of general and regional anesthetic may be utilized to provide both unconsciousness and pain relief. This strategy may be customized to meet your medical requirements and preferences, and your anesthesiologist will review the choices with you before surgery.

A Step-By-Step Overview Of The Surgical Procedure

Hip replacement surgery is a difficult process that consists of multiple phases, each of which is meticulously carried out by a qualified surgical team. Here's a summary of what to anticipate during the surgical procedure:

1. **Preparation:** Before the procedure, you will be transported to the operating room and seated on the operating table. Your surgical team will clean and sanitize the surgery site to limit the possibility of infection.

2. The surgeon will create an incision above the hip joint, usually along the side or front of the hip. The

size and location of the incision may vary depending on the surgical technique employed.

3. Damaged Tissue Removal: After making the incision, the surgeon will gently pull the muscles and other tissues aside to provide access to the hip joint. The injured or diseased hip joint components, including the damaged cartilage and bone, will be removed.

4. Implant placement: After removing the diseased tissue, the surgeon will prepare the remaining bone surfaces to accept the replacement hip components. These components, which may be composed of metal, plastic, or ceramic materials, are carefully chosen to match your body and perform optimally.

5. Closure: After the replacement hip components are installed, the surgeon will seal the incision with sutures or staples. A sterile bandage may be put on the incision site to improve healing and minimize the risk of infection.

Potential Risks And Complications

While hip replacement surgery is typically safe and successful, it does include certain risks and problems, as with any surgical operation. Before having surgery, you should discuss the risks with your surgeon. Some frequent dangers and consequences are:

1. Infection: Even with careful sterile methods, there is a danger of infection at the surgical site or in the deeper tissues around the hip joint. Infection symptoms include fever, increased discomfort, redness, and discharge from the incision site.

2. Blood Clots: Surgery and subsequent immobilization might raise the chance of blood clots forming in the legs, known as deep vein thrombosis (DVT), or spreading to the lungs, known as pulmonary embolism. To lessen this risk, your medical staff may provide blood thinners and promote early mobility.

3. **Dislocation:** In certain circumstances, the artificial hip joint may become dislocated, which means that the ball of the femoral component falls out of the socket. This may cause discomfort and instability, necessitating further surgery to resolve.

4. **Implant Wear and Loosening:** Over time, the prosthetic hip components may wear out or become loose, causing discomfort and reduced function. Revision surgery may be required to replace or repair the implants.

Post-Surgical Recovery In The Hospital

Following hip replacement surgery, you will be carefully observed in the hospital for many days to ensure your safety and comfort throughout the early stages of rehabilitation. Here's what to anticipate throughout this time:

1. **Pain Management:** Your medical staff will prescribe pain relievers to help you feel better after surgery. This might include oral drugs, intravenous (IV) pain treatment, or regional anesthesia procedures.

2. **Physical Therapy:** A physical therapist will work with you shortly after surgery to help you rebuild strength, flexibility, and mobility in your hip. This might include light exercises, walking with support equipment such as a walker or crutches, and learning suitable procedures for getting in and out of bed and chairs.

3. **Monitoring:** Your medical team will periodically check your vital signs, incision site, and general health to detect and treat any symptoms of problems, such as infection or blood clots.

4. **Diet and Hydration:** To promote recovery and avoid problems, remain hydrated and eat a well-balanced diet. Throughout your hospital stay, your healthcare

team will advise you on food limitations and hydration targets.

5. Discharge Planning: Before you leave the hospital, your medical team will work with you and your caregivers to facilitate a seamless transition to home. This may involve arranging for any required medical equipment or home care services, as well as giving instructions for wound care, medication management, and activity limits during the first stages of recuperation.

Overall, the post-surgery recovery phase at the hospital is crucial for healing and rehabilitation, and your medical team will be by your side every step of the way. By following their advice and actively participating in your rehabilitation, you may increase the success of your hip replacement surgery and experience greater mobility and quality of life in the long run.

CHAPTER 5

Post-Surgical Recovery

Pain Management Techniques

Managing pain following hip replacement surgery is critical for a healthy recovery. To assist reduce your agony, your medical staff may most likely prescribe pain medication. These might be over-the-counter pain remedies like ibuprofen or acetaminophen, or stronger prescription drugs if required. To successfully control pain while reducing the risk of adverse effects, you must take these drugs exactly as prescribed by your doctor.

In addition to medicine, there are other non-pharmacological pain treatment approaches to consider. Ice packs may help decrease inflammation and numb the surgery site, relieving discomfort. Just be sure to put a cloth or towel between the ice pack and your skin to avoid ice burn.

Warm baths or heating pads may also help relax muscles and relieve pain.

Relaxation methods such as deep breathing exercises, meditation, or guided imagery may assist in diverting from discomfort and induce calm. Physical therapy treatments such as mild stretching and massage may also help relieve muscular tension and discomfort.

It's important to be upfront with your medical staff about your pain levels and any concerns you may have. They may change your pain management strategy to keep you as comfortable as possible throughout your recovery.

Physical Therapy Exercises For Recovery

Physical therapy is essential in the rehabilitation process after hip replacement surgery. Your doctor will most likely suggest that you begin physical therapy shortly after surgery to help rebuild strength, flexibility, and range of motion in your hip joint.

Your physical therapist will create a customized workout program based on your requirements and skills. These exercises may include moderate stretching to increase flexibility, strengthening activities to rebuild muscle and range of motion exercises to restore hip joint mobility.

To get the greatest results, you must strictly adhere to your physical therapist's directions and execute your exercises consistently. While it is typical to feel some discomfort during physical therapy, it is critical to share with your therapist if you are experiencing severe pain or difficulties executing certain motions.

In addition to official physical therapy appointments, your therapist may offer home activities to augment your treatment. Simple exercises such as walking, cycling, or swimming may assist increase hip strength and mobility.

Consistency is essential in physical therapy. Stick to your fitness plan and don't become discouraged by failures or problems. With time and effort, you will gradually develop strength and mobility in your hip joint, enabling you to resume your typical activities more comfortably.

Managing Daily Activities Throughout Recovery

Recovery following hip replacement surgery requires patience and changes to your daily routine. While you may have some limits at first, there are various ways you may employ to manage your everyday tasks while recovering.

First and foremost, adhere to your doctor's advice for weight-bearing restrictions and activity limits. Avoid activities that place too much pressure on your hip joint, such as lifting heavy things or doing high-impact workouts.

Make changes to your living environment to promote a safe and pleasant recovery. This might involve adding handrails in the bathroom and near stairs, utilizing a shower chair or bath seat, and moving furniture to make clear routes for walking.

Take pauses during the day to recuperate and prevent overexertion. Listen to your body and pace yourself appropriately, gradually increasing your activity level as you recuperate.

Enlist the assistance of family members, friends, or caretakers to do duties that may be difficult during your recuperation time. Don't be afraid to ask for assistance when you need it, and speak honestly with others around you.

Finally, keep optimistic and focused on your rehabilitation objectives. Celebrate your success along the journey, and don't be disheartened by setbacks or challenges. With time and persistence, you will gradually recover your strength and independence, enabling you to confidently resume your daily activities.

Potential Complications And How To Manage Them

While hip replacement surgery is typically safe and successful, certain issues may arise during the recovery period. It is important to be aware of these issues and understand how to handle them if they emerge.

Infection at the surgery site is a typical complication. Infection may cause greater pain, edema, redness, or discharge from the incision site. If you feel you have an infection, call your doctor right away. Antibiotics may be used to treat the infection, or in extreme situations, surgical intervention to remove the affected tissue.

Another possible risk is blood clots, which may develop in your leg veins and spread to your lungs, resulting in pulmonary embolism.

To lower the risk of blood clots, your doctor may prescribe blood thinners, compression stockings, and leg exercises to improve circulation.

Dislocation of the hip joint is another potential consequence, especially in the early phases of rehabilitation. To limit the chance of dislocation, follow your doctor's recommendations for mobility restrictions and precautions. Avoid crossing your legs, bending your hips beyond a particular degree, or twisting your hip joint.

Nerve and blood artery damage are potentially possible consequences of hip replacement surgery. Symptoms of the afflicted leg may include numbness, tingling, weakness, or sensory alterations. If you encounter any of these symptoms, contact your doctor right away for additional assessment and treatment.

Being aware of possible issues and making early efforts to address them may help you reduce the risk of difficulties and ensure a safe and successful recovery following hip replacement surgery. Make sure to strictly follow your doctor's advice and discuss any concerns or symptoms you may have throughout your recuperation.

CHAPTER 6

Rehabilitation And Physical Therapy

Importance Of Rehabilitation Following Hip Replacement Surgery

Rehabilitation after hip replacement surgery is critical for a good recovery and restoring mobility and function to the hip joint. This phase of therapy helps patients rebuild hip strength, flexibility, and range of motion while also improving general physical fitness and quality of life.

Patients may have pain, discomfort, and stiffness in the hip joint immediately after surgery. Rehabilitation reduces these symptoms and aids recovery by gradually increasing exercise and restoring normal movement patterns.

Participating in an organized rehabilitation program under the supervision of a physical therapist helps patients recover confidence in utilizing their new hip joint and lowers the risk of problems such as muscle weakness, joint stiffness, and instability.

Throughout the rehabilitation process, patients are taught suitable strategies for walking, climbing stairs, and doing everyday tasks to guarantee optimum function and avoid damage.

Regular involvement in rehabilitation exercises also aids in the prevention of muscle atrophy and joint stiffness, both of which may arise if the hip joint is not moved appropriately throughout the healing period.

Patients who concentrate on rehabilitation following hip replacement surgery may obtain better results and return to regular activities with more comfort and mobility.

Schedule For Rehabilitation Exercises

The timing of rehabilitation activities after hip replacement surgery varies depending on the amount of the operation, the patient's general health, and any pre-existing medical issues. However, most patients see a general progression as they recuperate following surgery.

Patients are urged to begin with a mild range of motion exercises in the early postoperative period to avoid stiffness and enhance circulation in the hip joint. These might include ankle pumps, heel slides, and moderate hip stretches done while reclining in bed.

As the discomfort and edema subside, patients often graduate to more advanced activities that improve hip joint strength, balance, and flexibility. Leg lifts, hip abduction and adduction movements, and mild stretching exercises may all help increase the range of motion.

By the second week following surgery, most patients can walk with the use of a walker or crutches. As patients' strength and confidence improve, they may progressively increase the distance and length of their walks, ultimately moving to walking independently.

By the sixth week following surgery, many patients may resume more demanding activities including swimming, cycling, and low-impact aerobics. However, it is critical to avoid high-impact sports like running and leaping until the hip joint has completely healed, which might take many months.

Patients should work closely with their physical therapist throughout the rehabilitation process to monitor their progress and adapt their exercise regimen as necessary. It is critical to follow the advice of the healthcare staff and avoid pushing too hard since this might result in setbacks and delays in recovery.

Exercises To Increase Strength And Mobility

Several workouts may help you regain strength and mobility following hip replacement surgery. These exercises increase stability and function by focusing on the muscles around the hip joint, as well as the core and lower extremities.

1. Hip Flexion: Sit on a chair with your feet flat on the floor. Slowly elevate your surgical leg off the ground, bending your knee and bringing it closer to your chest. Hold for a few seconds and then drop your leg back down. Repeat 10–15 times on each leg.

2. Hip Extension: For support, stand behind a solid chair or countertop. Slowly raise your surgical leg backward while maintaining your knee straight. Hold for a few seconds and then drop your leg back down. Repeat 10–15 times on each leg.

3. Hip abduction: Lie on your non-surgical side, legs straight. Lift your surgical leg, maintaining it straight, and then drop it back down. Repeat 10–15 times on each leg.

4. Hip Adduction: Lie on your back, knees bent, feet flat on the floor. Put a cushion between your knees. Squeeze your knees together to engage the inner thigh muscles, then relax. Repeat 10 to 15 times.

5. Quadriceps Strengthening: Sit on the edge of a chair and stretch your surgical leg in front of you. Tighten the muscles at the front of your thighs and raise your leg off the ground, straightening your knee. Hold for a few seconds and then drop your leg back down. Repeat 10–15 times on each leg.

6. Core Strengthening: Exercises such as pelvic tilts, abdominal bracing, and leg lifts may help strengthen the core muscles, which offer stability and support to the hip joint.

To increase hip joint strength, flexibility, and mobility, executes these exercises regularly as part of a complete rehabilitation program.

Tips For A Successful Rehabilitation Process

1. Follow the Rehabilitation Program: Attend all planned physical therapy appointments and adhere to the exercise plan given by your healthcare provider. Consistency is essential for attaining the best outcomes.

2. Take it Slow: Pay attention to your body and build up your fitness routine gradually. Avoid pushing through pain or discomfort since it might result in harm or setbacks in your recovery.

3. Stay Active: Walking, swimming, and cycling are all low-impact activities that may help you maintain your cardiovascular fitness and general health while you recuperate.

4. Use Assistive Devices as Needed: During the early stages of rehabilitation, your healthcare provider may suggest using a walker, cane, or crutches to help you walk and avoid falls.

5. Practice Good Posture and Body Mechanics: Pay attention to your posture and body mechanics while doing everyday tasks to decrease pressure on the hip joint and avoid injury.

6. Maintain a positive attitude: Recovering following hip replacement surgery requires time and patience. Stay optimistic and focused on your objectives, and appreciate tiny triumphs along the way.

By following these guidelines and adhering to your rehabilitation program, you may recover successfully and resume your daily activities with better hip joint mobility and function.

CHAPTER 7

Returning To Daily Activities

Gradual Resumption Of Daily Activity

Returning to normal activities after hip replacement surgery is an important element of the rehabilitation process. However, to promote adequate healing and avoid difficulties, this should be done gradually and cautiously. Your healthcare team will advise you on when it is safe to resume specific activities depending on your unique recovery and the kind of surgery you had.

In the days immediately after surgery, you may want help with simple chores such as showering, dressing, and getting in and out of bed. As your strength and mobility improve, you may progressively ramp up your exercise level. It's important to listen to your body and prevent overexertion since pushing yourself too hard too soon might cause delays in your recovery.

Modifications For Activities Such As Driving And Household Chores

Certain tasks, including driving and housework, may need to be modified temporarily to allow your rehabilitation. Driving, for example, may be prohibited for some time after surgery, usually until you are no longer using pain medicines and can safely drive a car. Your surgeon will advise you on when it is safe to start driving depending on your specific situation.

Household duties may also be changed to reduce stress on your hip joint during the first stages of recuperation. This may include utilizing assistive equipment like a reacher or long-handled sponge to minimize bending or twisting, which may place strain on the hip. Simple adaptations, such as utilizing a shower chair or a higher toilet seat, may help you handle these duties while regaining strength and mobility.

Guidelines For Physical Activity And Exercise

Physical activity and exercise are critical for your long-term rehabilitation and the success of hip replacement surgery. Your healthcare provider will make specific suggestions depending on your condition and fitness level, but in general, stretching, strengthening, and cardiovascular workouts are good.

Low-impact sports like walking, swimming, and cycling are ideal for increasing joint flexibility and muscular strength without placing too much strain on the hip joint. Gentle stretching exercises may assist preserve flexibility, but resistance training with modest weights or resistance bands can help develop muscle around the hip joint to provide additional support.

Long-Term Expectations For Hip Function

While the primary objective of hip replacement surgery is to alleviate pain and enhance mobility, it is critical to set reasonable expectations for long-term hip function. Most patients see a considerable improvement in pain and movement after surgery, enabling them to resume many of their favorite activities.

However, it is critical to recognize that hip replacement surgery does not fully return the joint to its previous state, and certain limits may remain. To minimize excessive wear on the artificial joint, avoid activities that entail high-impact or repeated movements, such as running or jumping.

You may enhance your long-term hip function and live an active lifestyle with less pain and more mobility by following your healthcare team's post-operative care recommendations, which include rehabilitation exercises and activity changes.

CHAPTER 8

Complications And Risks

Common Complications Following Hip Replacement Surgery

Hip replacement surgery is typically safe and effective, but as with any surgical operation, there are risks and problems to consider. Understanding these issues may help patients and caregivers plan for their recovery and identify when they need to seek medical assistance.

Infection is a frequent complication after hip replacement surgery. Although infections are uncommon, they may develop at the surgical site or in the deeper tissues around the hip joint. Infection symptoms may include increasing pain, edema, redness, warmth, or discharge from the incision site. In certain situations, individuals may develop a fever. Prompt antibiotic therapy is critical to preventing infection spread and minimizing harm to the replacement hip joint.

Another possible consequence is hip dislocation. This happens when the ball of the artificial joint is displaced from its socket. Patients are often advised to take specific measures, such as avoiding certain motions and postures, to limit the chance of dislocation during the early healing phase. Despite these safeguards, dislocation may still occur, particularly if patients fail to follow their postoperative instructions.

In addition to infection and dislocation, potential risks of hip replacement surgery include blood clots, nerve damage, and implant failure. Deep vein thrombosis (DVT) is a disorder in which blood clots develop in the veins of the legs and may migrate to the lungs, resulting in a pulmonary embolism. Patients may be prescribed blood-thinning drugs as well as instructions to wear compression stockings and practice leg exercises to avoid blood clots.

Nerve damage is another possible risk of hip replacement surgery, albeit it is uncommon. Nerve injury may result in numbness, weakness, or discomfort in the afflicted limb, and in extreme instances, lifelong impairment. Careful surgical technique and thorough postoperative care may reduce the chance of nerve damage.

Implant failure is an uncommon but dangerous problem that may need revision surgery to resolve. Implant failure may be caused by a variety of causes, including component loosening, wear of the prosthetic joint surfaces, and bone fracture surrounding the implant. Regular follow-up meetings with the surgeon, as well as periodic imaging scans, may aid in the early detection of implant issues and the prevention of future difficulties.

Overall, although complications following hip replacement surgery are infrequent, patients must be aware of the signs and symptoms of possible difficulties and seek immediate medical assistance if they arise. Patients who follow their surgeon's recommendations and participate fully in their rehabilitation may lessen the risk of problems and reap the advantages of a successful hip replacement surgery.

Symptoms Of An Infection Or Other Complications

Monitoring for symptoms of infection or other issues after hip replacement surgery is critical to ensuring early management and the best results. While problems are uncommon, being aware of possible warning signals may help patients and caregivers respond quickly if they emerge.

Increased pain, swelling, redness, or warmth at the surgical site is a common indicator of infection. These symptoms might signal that the body is establishing an immunological response to microorganisms introduced during surgery. Additionally, leakage from the incision site, especially if it is yellow, green, or foul-smelling, might be an indication of infection. Patients should also be aware of indicators of systemic illness, such as fever, chills, and malaise.

In addition to infection, various complications of hip replacement surgery may cause distinct symptoms. For example, hip joint dislocation may result in abrupt, intense discomfort and the inability to bear weight on the afflicted limb. Patients may also feel a popping or clicking feeling in their hip joint. Another possible risk is blood clots, which may cause swelling, soreness, and warmth in the afflicted leg, as well as redness or coloring of skin.

Another risk is nerve damage, which may cause symptoms such as numbness, tingling, weakness, or pain in the legs or feet. Patients should notify their healthcare physician right away if they have any strange symptoms or sensory changes. While implant failure is less frequent, symptoms may include increasing discomfort, joint instability or looseness, or a reduction in range of motion.

If patients develop any of these signs or symptoms following hip replacement surgery, they should call their surgeon or seek medical assistance immediately. Early intervention may help prevent issues from escalating and increase the likelihood of a good result. In rare circumstances, immediate treatment may be required to avoid severe consequences or lasting harm.

Steps To Take If Complications Arise

If issues emerge after hip replacement surgery, immediate treatment is required to manage them and prevent possible injury. Patients and caregivers should be prepared to take particular actions to promote the greatest possible result and recovery.

The first step in dealing with difficulties is to call the surgeon or healthcare professional who conducted the hip replacement surgery. They are knowledgeable about the patient's medical history and may provide individualized advice depending on the type and severity of the issue. Patients should be ready to explain their symptoms in detail and offer any pertinent information, such as changes in medication or activity level.

In certain circumstances, the surgeon may suggest conservative treatments to treat the problem, such as rest, ice, elevation, or pain medication. For more significant issues, such as infection or implant failure, further procedures may be required. This may involve antibiotics, fluid or pus discharge from the surgical site, or revision surgery to repair or replace the implant.

Patients should also follow their healthcare provider's recommendations for wound care, activity limits, and follow-up consultations.

To maximize recovery and reduce the risk of problems, please follow these directions. Patients may also be sent to experts in infectious illness or physical therapy for further examination and treatment.

Throughout the rehabilitation process, open contact with the healthcare staff is essential. Patients should feel free to ask questions, voice concerns, and seek clarity on their treatment plans. Patients may increase their chances of success and return to an active, pain-free lifestyle by collaborating closely with their healthcare doctors and according to their suggestions.

Strategies To Prevent Complications

While problems following hip replacement surgery cannot always be completely avoided, patients and healthcare professionals may use a variety of techniques to lower the risk and encourage the best possible results. Patients may reduce the risk of problems and ensure a smooth recovery by adopting proactive actions before, during, and after surgery.

Preoperative optimization is critical for lowering the likelihood of problems after hip replacement surgery. This may entail treating underlying medical disorders, such as diabetes or high blood pressure, which may raise the risk of surgical complications. Patients may be urged to stop smoking, reduce weight, or change their diet to increase their general health and healing capability.

During the surgical operation, paying close attention to technique and surgeon competence may help reduce the risk of problems including infection, nerve damage, or implant malposition. Surgeons may use specific methods, such as antibiotic-coated implants or less invasive procedures, to lower the risk of infection and encourage speedier healing.

Postoperative care is very important in avoiding problems after hip replacement surgery. Patients should closely follow their surgeon's recommendations for wound care, activity limits, and medication management. Physical therapy and rehabilitation activities are essential for restoring strength, flexibility, and function to the hip joint while lowering the risk of problems like stiffness or muscle weakness.

In addition to these strategies, patients may improve their general health and well-being by keeping a healthy weight, being physically active, and treating chronic medical illnesses. Regular follow-up meetings with the surgeon and other healthcare specialists may help spot any difficulties early on and respond quickly to avoid future problems.

Patients who take a proactive approach to prevention and rehabilitation may reduce their risk of problems following hip replacement surgery and obtain the best potential result. Open communication with the healthcare staff, following postoperative instructions, and committing to self-care are all necessary components of a successful recovery.

CHAPTER 9

Lifestyle Modifications Recommendations To Maintain Hip Health

Maintaining hip health is critical for those who have had hip replacement surgery and those who wish to avoid hip issues in the future. Several lifestyle changes may dramatically improve hip health and general well-being.

First and foremost, a healthy weight must be maintained. Excess weight increases stress on the hip joints, possibly speeding up wear and tear. Individuals who maintain a healthy weight via a balanced diet and regular exercise may lessen stress on their hips and enhance overall joint function.

Second, practicing proper posture is essential. Poor posture may result in hip misalignment, which causes pain and increases the risk of injury. Individuals who maintain good alignment and posture may lessen pressure on their hip joints and increase overall joint health.

Furthermore, avoiding high-impact sports might help prevent the hip joints from premature wear and strain. Running and leaping may place too much stress on the hips, causing joint injury over time. Individuals can instead concentrate on low-impact workouts like swimming, cycling, or walking to keep their hips healthy without placing too much pressure on the joints.

Finally, listen to your body and notice any indicators of discomfort or pain. Ignoring pain or pushing through discomfort might result in severe hip joint damage and degradation. Listening to your body and resolving any abnormalities as soon as possible can help you maintain optimum hip health and avoid future problems.

Dietary Considerations For Bone Health

A well-balanced diet is essential for keeping strong and healthy bones, especially the hips. Several critical nutrients are necessary for bone health and may aid in the recovery process after hip replacement surgery.

For starters, calcium is essential for the formation and maintenance of healthy bones. Calcium-rich foods include milk, cheese, and yogurt, as well as leafy greens like kale and spinach. Incorporating these calcium-rich foods into your diet will assist with bone health and the healing process after hip replacement surgery.

Second, vitamin D is required for calcium absorption and contributes significantly to bone health. Vitamin D may be found in fatty fish like salmon and tuna, egg yolks, and fortified foods like milk and orange juice. Additionally, spending time outside in the sun might help your body create vitamin D naturally.

Furthermore, protein is necessary for bone health and might aid in the recovery process after surgery. Incorporating lean protein sources into your diet, such as chicken, fish, beans, and nuts, may help support bone health and healing.

Finally, keeping hydrated is important for general health and may aid in the recovery process after hip replacement surgery. Drinking enough water every day might help keep your bones and joints lubricated and working correctly.

Exercise And Activity Guidelines For Long-Term Hip Health

Regular exercise and physical activity are critical for preserving long-term hip health and general well-being. However, it is critical to choose activities that are safe and acceptable for those who have had hip replacement surgery.

Low-impact workouts like swimming, cycling, and walking are great for improving hip health without placing too much load on the joints. These exercises promote flexibility, strength, and cardiovascular fitness while minimizing hip joint injury.

Stretching exercises may also assist increase hip flexibility and range of motion, lowering the risk of injury and increasing overall joint function. Including simple stretching exercises in your everyday routine will help keep your hips flexible and mobile.

Strength training routines are necessary to maintain muscle strength and stability around the hip joints. However, it is critical to begin with small weights and gradually build intensity to prevent placing too much pressure on the freshly restored joint. Working with a physical therapist or personal trainer may help you create a safe and effective strength training program that is personalized to your specific requirements.

Furthermore, exercising proper posture and body mechanics throughout everyday tasks might assist in lessening stress on the hip joints and avoid injury. Avoiding activities that involve extensive bending or twisting of the hips may help preserve the joints and maintain long-term hip health.

Tips To Prevent Future Hip Problems

Preventing future hip issues requires a proactive approach to total joint health and wellness. In addition to the advice listed above, numerous more measures may help lower the likelihood of hip issues in the future.

First and foremost, it is important to maintain a healthy lifestyle. This involves eating a well-balanced diet, exercising frequently, staying at a healthy weight, and refraining from smoking and drinking excessively. These lifestyle behaviors may all help to improve overall joint health and lower the chance of hip issues.

Second, keeping your hips from damage is critical. This includes avoiding activities that place too much pressure on the hips, wearing suitable footwear, and using optimal body mechanics while lifting or moving large things. Preventing injury may help protect your hips and lessen the chance of future issues.

Furthermore, keeping active and participating in regular physical exercise is critical for hip health and general well-being. Incorporating a range of low-impact exercises into your program will help strengthen the muscles surrounding your hips, increase flexibility, and lower your risk of injury.

Finally, being aware of your hip health and swiftly addressing any worries or difficulties might help avoid future problems. If you have chronic hip pain, discomfort, or other symptoms, you should visit with a healthcare expert to get an exact diagnosis and treatment.

By making proactive efforts to safeguard your hip health, you may lower your risk of future issues and maintain a healthy and active lifestyle for years to come.

CHAPTER 10
Moving Forward

Recap Of Key Points On Hip Replacement Surgery

Hip replacement surgery is a life-changing technique that relieves pain and improves movement in those who have significant hip joint degeneration. This handbook has covered a variety of topics, from preoperative preparations to postoperative care. Let's go over some crucial elements to guarantee a thorough comprehension.

Understanding the Surgery: Hip replacement surgery is replacing the injured hip joint with an artificial one composed of metal, plastic, or ceramic materials. This surgery seeks to restore hip joint function while also alleviating pain caused by disorders such as arthritis or fracture.

Preoperative Preparations: Before surgery, patients go through a series of assessments, which include physical exams, imaging tests, and conversations about their medical history and possible hazards. Preparing emotionally and physically for surgery is critical for a good result.

Surgical Procedure: The orthopedic surgeon creates an incision to get access to the hip joint. The damaged bone and cartilage are removed, and the artificial implant is firmly fixed in place. The surgical team ensures that the implant is precisely aligned and stable for maximum performance.

Postoperative Care: Following surgery, patients are continuously followed in the hospital for problems. Pain management, rehabilitation activities, and measures against dislocation are critical throughout the healing period. Physical therapy may help you restore strength and mobility in your hip joint.

Potential Risks and Complications: While hip replacement surgery is typically safe, there are certain risks, including infection, blood clotting, implant displacement, and nerve injury. Following postoperative instructions and attending follow-up consultations may assist in reducing these risks.

Encouragement To Continue Recovery And Rehabilitation

Recovery following hip replacement surgery is a long process that involves patience, commitment, and effort. It is critical to remain motivated and devoted to the rehabilitation regimen prescribed by your healthcare team.

Stay Active: Regular physical exercise is essential for maintaining the strength and flexibility of the hip joint. Your physical therapist will walk you through the proper exercises to enhance mobility and avoid stiffness.

Follow Medical Advice: Schedule follow-up visits with your orthopedic surgeon and other healthcare experts. They will track your progress, address any issues, and modify your treatment plan as required to guarantee your full recovery.

Manage Expectations: It is typical to feel some pain and limits in the early stages of rehabilitation. Be patient with yourself and concentrate on minor accomplishments along the road. With time and effort, you'll gradually recover mobility and return to your normal activities.

Seek help: If you need emotional help throughout your rehabilitation, don't be afraid to contact family members, friends, or support groups. Sharing your thoughts and worries with people who have gone through similar treatments may be helpful and empowering.

Looking Ahead: Life Following Hip Replacement Surgery

Hip replacement surgery gives many people a new lease on life, enabling them to experience more mobility, less discomfort, and a higher quality of life. As you continue through the rehabilitation process, it's crucial to look forward and imagine the possibilities that await.

Regaining Independence: With the help of your healthcare team and loved ones, you may gradually recover independence and autonomy in your everyday activities. Simple actions like walking, climbing stairs, and getting in and out of chairs will grow simpler with time.

Returning to Activities: As your hip joint strengthens and recovers, you will be able to gradually resume activities you like, such as gardening, swimming, and sports. It's critical to listen to your body and prevent overexertion, particularly in the early phases of recuperation.

Embracing a Healthy Lifestyle: Hip replacement surgery may spark good lifestyle changes. Adopting a good diet, keeping a healthy weight, and quitting smoking may all contribute to the long-term effectiveness of your hip replacement while also improving your general health and well-being.

Staying Informed: Stay up to date on improvements in hip replacement technology and methods. Your orthopedic surgeon can advise you on the newest advancements and treatments that may help you in the future.

Enjoying Life: Finally, hip replacement surgery is about recovering your quality of life and engaging in things that offer you pleasure and satisfaction. By taking proactive actions to care for your hip joint and general health, you may look forward to a life full of mobility, energy, and enjoyment.

Conclusion

To summarize, hip replacement surgery is a revolutionary treatment that may greatly enhance the quality of life for anyone suffering from painful hip disorders such as osteoarthritis, rheumatoid arthritis, or hip fractures. Throughout this book, we've covered everything from hip replacement surgery indications and preparation to the surgical operation itself, recuperation, and possible problems.

Understanding the indications for hip replacement surgery is critical. Patients with significant pain, stiffness, and limited mobility owing to hip joint degeneration or injury are often candidates for this therapy. Patients may restore mobility and reduce discomfort by replacing the injured joint with an artificial implant, enabling them to resume their everyday activities in greater comfort and usefulness.

Hip replacement surgery requires a full medical examination, including diagnostic testing and evaluations, to ensure that patients are physically and psychologically prepared for the treatment. In addition, patients may need to adopt lifestyle changes, such as stopping smoking or decreasing weight, to improve surgery results and lower the chance of complications.

The surgical treatment consists of removing damaged hip joint components and replacing them with artificial components composed of metal, plastic, or ceramic materials. Surgeons use a variety of procedures, including standard hip replacement and minimally invasive alternatives, to execute the operation with accuracy and reduce tissue damage. Advances in surgical equipment and procedures continue to improve results, making shorter hospital stays and quicker recovery periods increasingly prevalent.

Recovery following hip replacement surgery is a long process that involves patience and dedication from both patients and healthcare professionals. Physical therapy is essential in restoring strength, flexibility, and mobility to the hip joint, enabling patients to eventually resume regular activities. While most patients see considerable improvements in pain and function after surgery, it is critical to follow post-operative instructions and attend follow-up sessions to evaluate progress and address any issues.

Despite the great success of hip replacement surgery, problems may arise, including infection, blood clots, implant displacement, and joint instability. However, by carefully selecting patients, using excellent surgical techniques, and providing extensive post-operative care, the risk of problems may be reduced while increasing the advantages of hip replacement surgery.

In conclusion, hip replacement surgery is a very successful therapeutic option for those suffering from severe hip joint difficulties. Understanding the indications, preparation, operation, recovery, and potential consequences of this surgery allows patients to make educated choices and collaborate with their healthcare professionals to obtain the best possible results and reclaim their quality of life.

THE END

www.ingramcontent.com/pod-product-compliance
Lightning Source LLC
Chambersburg PA
CBHW071838210526
45479CB00001B/194